F _ _ _ Him!

when, where, how

by velicia hill

This book is dedicated to him...

Many thanks to all my girlfriends that I forced to read my early drafts...drinks are on me. But most of all, to my talented & PATIENT copy editor, Jane Garretson, my very own grammar cop. Without you this book would not be possible...or it would be a hot grammatical mess—THANK YOU!

Table of Contents

I. INTRODUCTION

II. WARNING

III. CAUTION

IV. NOTICE

V. Handling & Usage

STEP #1: F _ _ _ HIM (well)!

STEP #2: F _ _ _ HIM (up)!

STEP #3: F _ _ _ HIM (often)!

STEP #4: F _ _ _ HIM (anywhere)!

STEP #5: F _ _ _ HIM (daily)!

STEP #6: F _ _ _ HIM (whenever)!

STEP #7: F _ _ _ HIM (quickly)!

BONUS TIP: F _ _ _ HIM (never)!

READ

ALL INSTRUCTIONS BEFORE USE!

INTRODUCTION

You're probably thinking, *"Why* do I need a book on how to f_ _ _ my man? I've been having sex since high school." Well, even if you've been spreading the love since the 80s, simply ask yourself these questions:

- Would you much rather scroll through social media than make love?
- Does your man joke to friends & family about sex-or lack thereof he gets from you?
- Do you need a cocktail before sex?
- Do you control every aspect of your relationship?
- Has your relationship experienced infidelity?
- Are you a missionary mama? Also known as a pillow princess!
- Do you enjoy your kids more than your mate?
- Do you fake sleep, pain or fatigue to avoid intimacy?

- Do you and your spouse/partner fight more than three times a month?

- Is sex reserved for birthdays (his), Father's Day, New Year's Eve and wedding anniversaries?

- Do you refer to him as your "other child?"

- Have you stopped kissing? And no, not that side cheek crap; but tongue kissing?

If you answered yes to any of these questions, then I hate to inform you-you need some new direction and instructions on how to f_ _ _ yo man!

I wrote this book in the manner of an instructional guide, like the instructions you'd find enclosed inside any electronic device. Matter of fact, I simply copied the instruction format that I found in my battery-operated fabric shaver & lint remover that I picked up from Walgreen's, right before I started writing this book.

Who gon check me, boo?

You!

I know you girls and boys so well; you've probably already *Googled* me and checked my credentials. Because you all HATE taking advice from someone who's never been in your wedding shoes. Well, I have. And yes, I did everything wrong for staying and maintaining a healthy marriage—hence my subsequent divorce. What's more, I'm not a doctor nor do I play one on T.V. My experience and expertise derive from a lot of dating, one marriage, one divorce and four called-off engagements. Trust me, I can navigate my way around the bedroom.

Unfortunately, I'm hardheaded. I like to learn the hard way. And therefore, I graduated with honors from the school of hard knocks.

And as the late great Maya Angelou said: *"When you learn, teach."*

As I type this on my computer, I'm single and dating. Hoping to one day find my prince charming and ride out in a beautiful Aston Martin, chasing a rainbow and a hot pink sunset, to the soft sounds of a certain 70s love song.

Let's face it-love is grand!

I know that nothing lasts forever; some people come into our lives for a season, others for a reason. But If you're going to do your best to be fully present in your union, I'm adding my take-no-prisoners two cents to an already heaping pile of advice I'm sure you've already received. And if he decides to leave and/or cheat, not knowing how to f_ _ _ him, won't be the reason why.

I still believe in the institution of marriage. There's nothing sexier and more heartwarming than when a man decides, that with all the women in the world (over 3.8 billion of us), that it is YOU that he wants to love for a lifetime! If that doesn't make your heart skip a beat-check your pulse! But even if you no longer believe in traditional marriage and prefer to just live with him, or if you're married to someone of the same sex, you can still benefit from these instructions. These instructions are simply about loving your mate (from a straight woman's point of view). This is not a how-to-get-married book. This advice is how-to-STAY married. But I am pretty confident that if you implement these tips while dating, you just might snag his ass.

Lastly, I'm willing to bet that no one has ever broken down the steps and instructions to f_ _ _ ing your man—not even your mother. And if she did, that's a rare woke woman- consider yourself very lucky.

At the minimum, sex education is taught in schools the last time I checked; but not *sexual* education- and yes, being sexual is a whole other subject.

Understanding how to really make love to the opposite sex isn't a course available at any public school or even at your local community center.

Seriously, what the hell people...do any of us, young or old, male or female, know what the f_ _ _ we're doing?

No wonder most of us don't know our clitoris from our vulva.

Yet we expect men to be master lovers and make us achieve multiple orgasms, when we can't even do it ourselves! If you're like me, you learned about sex from friends, porn, television, books, online and good ole trial and error. Well, fret no more; I've done the legs (in the air) work for you and after reading these instructions and putting them into use, you will be a helluva lover and know exactly how to f _ _ _ him!

WARNING:

YOU MUST MARRY A MAN YOU RESPECT MUCH MORE THAN YOU LOVE!

YOU MUST MARRY A MAN YOU RESPECT MUCH MORE THAN YOU LOVE!

YOU MUST MARRY A MAN YOU RESPECT MUCH MORE THAN YOU LOVE!

YOU MUST MARRY A MAN YOU RESPECT MUCH MORE THAN YOU LOVE!

YOU MUST MARRY A MAN YOU RESPECT MUCH MORE THAN YOU LOVE!

YOU MUST MARRY A MAN YOU RESPECT MUCH MORE THAN YOU LOVE!

Please re-read that sentence like ten more times; because ain't NONE of these instructions will work if you do not hook up with a guy whom you absolutely adore! All while respecting his brain, his hustle, his courage, his style (or lack thereof), and anything that makes him, him.

Respect is just a fancier word for like. You must *really* like the man you're marrying.

And if you don't like him, his teeth, his smile, his

height, his breathing patterns (that asinine in & out), his business skills, then DO NOT WALK YO ASS DOWN THAT AISLE! That was my mistake: I MARRIED A MAN I LOVED. BUT (and this is huge), I DIDN'T MARRY A MAN I

TRULY RESPECTED...IN TURN--LIKED!

- Marry your friend.
- Marry a man with whom you can be completely yourself.
- Marry someone you really enjoy hanging out with.
- Marry a man that you trust.
- Marry a man that will honor and respect your past...including your mistakes, bad decisions, and your "ancient" whore tendencies.
- Marry a man that doesn't try to control you.
- Marry a man that you can freely share your future hopes and dreams with.
- Marry a man that challenges you and calls you out on your shit.
- Marry a man that makes you laugh.

My only reason for divulging this much information gratuitously (as you'll see), is for you to learn from me.

So, let me reiterate, I did not respect (LIKE) my ex-husband and in turn, after a while,

I did not

like him,

nor

his kisses on the mouth.

Or sex WITHOUT alcohol...yep, I just said it—OUT LOUD...sip on that! I will go more in depth on this salacious, underdiscussed subject later.

CAUTION:

To reduce the risk of harming yourself or others-

Do not marry, date/engage with a man, out of loneliness or fear of being alone.

Do not ignore disturbing behavior, hobbies or interests.

Do not fake orgasms.

NOTICE:

To reduce the risk of damage to this book and/or yourself-

Do not read with a closed mind.

Do not share with girlfriends; make them get their own copy.

Do not try to convince those that disagree with the enclosed instructions.

Do not read at church, nunneries, or anyplace that suppresses a woman's sexual aptitude.

Do not skip or flip ahead-READ IT FROM THE BEGINNING!

Handling & Usage:

FOR ADULTS ONLY.

Intended for those over 18

Keep away from children and preteens.

Did you read <u>ALL</u> instructions??? The instructions are like foreplay… it's better when you take your time.

STEP #1

F <u>e e d</u> HIM!

> *"Food is symbolic of love when words are inadequate."*
>
> *~A. Ian D. Wolfelt*

Aha...*gotcha!* You thought this was like so many first dates, straight to the bedroom—NOPE! We're NOT starting with what you put in your mouth, but in *his*—food!

What's for dinner?

Reservations...NOT!

I'm sure you've heard the cliché, "The fastest way to a man's heart is through his stomach." Well, it's true. Men love to eat.

Pure and simple.

That's why you must get on the fast track, in the kitchen, and start to cook.

Why cook?

Because it will remind him of being a little boy (and never forget, your grown-ass man will always be a little boy at heart). When you cook for him, it'll remind him of how his mommy would cook, cut up and make sure his food was the perfect temperature. Now I'm not saying cut up his food, blow on it and feed it to him; but what I am saying is, that if you cook, it will stoke an old, fond, familiar, memory of endearment for him.

Why?

Food is love.

"There is no sight on earth more appealing than the sight of a woman making dinner for someone she loves."

~Thomas Wolfe

And yes, I can hear the collective groans and see the head rolls all the way over here from my neck of the woods. But even if you can't cook, do a semi-homemade meal. You can go to any store or restaurant and get some portion of your meal prepared by someone else, backed up by your specialty.

And I'm willing to bet you have a specialty or two left over from your days of being a single chick.

Moreover, I'm well aware that this is something

you probably won't be able to do every day, if you also work outside the home. But whenever you can, please cook and bake something-IF, you want a stronger union.

Wanna know why people love their mom's or grandmother's cooking?

Because the secret ingredient is...wait for it: LOVE!

"Everything important I learned, I learned as a dishwasher."

~Anthony Bourdain

I feel as if I can discern your thoughts right now. There are some of you out there telling me, okay, more like *yelling* at me, that you don't cook--your husband is the cook in the house.

I feel ya, girl. BUT...I'm still not letting you off the hook just yet.

If your husband is the Benny Crocker of the house, then I need you to follow Anthony Bourdain's lead and become the best damn unpaid dishwasher—you got some serious lessons to learn!

In its essence, what Anthony is saying, by washing dishes he learned order.

Every successful restaurant is run by good order.

It takes teamwork to make the dream work.

It doesn't matter if the tastiest food with the best organic ingredients is being prepared, it won't mean a damn thang, if it's not being served on clean plates accompanied by spotless silverware.

Thereupon, there really isn't any one position in the kitchen that's more important or paramount in the hierarchy. Of course, the dishwasher is the lowest on the totem pole and the chef gets all the glory; but let a food inspector make an unplanned visit to a filthy, unsanitary kitchen and the *entire* restaurant well get a failing score!

Your home should follow suit.

Rethink your role in the kitchen.

Do the damn dishes.

STEP #2

F <u>u</u> <u>e</u> <u>l</u> HIM!

"Love, like fire, goes out without fuel."

~ Mikhail Lermontov

Man Does Not Live by Bread Alone

Translation: feed your man's soul.

They don't call it soul food for nothing!

"You are the butter to my bread, and the breath to my life" ~ Julia Child

Talk to him and really listen to what he has to say.

PUT DOWN THAT DAMN CELL PHONE!

Make and maintain eye contact.

There's nothing sexier than looking your man directly in his eyes and really seeing him for exactly who he is.

And there's nothing worse than seeing a couple out to dinner with nothing to converse about sitting there bored, staring at other couples, critiquing single girls' wardrobes, or each on their individual cell phones.

"You can't fake listening. It shows." ~Raquel Welch

If you find yourself constantly on your phone, you need to ask yourself why playing *CandyCrush* or gossiping for hours with your bestie, *or* scrollin' Instagram every ten minutes is so much more fun than playing with your mate?

Really???

I'm not saying never have a two-hour gab fest with your girls, but when he first comes home, give him your undivided attention.

Especially when he's been working all day, he will need a decompress partner:

- Someone he can share his day with.
- Someone to tell him everything's gon be alright.
- Someone to greet him warmly after a long day.

"Home is where someone runs to greet you." ~Unknown

Matter of fact, you and your dog should be running and competing to see who gets to the door first!

(I see your bulging eyes)

Whatever girl, you better beat that bitch to the door- it works!

Additionally, I can always tell when a couple is in a marriage that's not wholly fulfilling.

What are the telltale signs you ask?

He or she is constantly posting online. Their social media presence is much too active for someone with a boo thang (I will excuse those that are social influencers). And yet, with all that activity, they rarely post pics of their spouse. Trust me, a lot of shit goes down in those DMs! I cannot begin to tell you how many married or boo'ed up men have crept into my DMs! Honestly, is *anybody* really happy? I'm starting to have my doubts.

Other signs

- one partner spends an inordinate amount of time away from the other.
- Dinners alone
- Separate bedtimes
- Numerous monthly business trips (accompanied by times when he's completely unreachable and phone calls go unanswered)

- Excessive activities with the children or inviting them to sleep in the master bedroom (they act as cockblockers)
- Too many late nights spent with other people

"Affairs don't start in bedrooms, they start with conversations."

~ Unknown

High Octane Fuel Only

Frequently keep him full with positive words of encouragement and flowery compliments. You're his forever girl; be gluttonous with your words.

Give him a nickname.

Treat him like an expensive Italian sports car; no regular fuel.

Oh no, baby boy gets the premium treatment! Keeps him from pinging and knocking (ladies, that's engine jargon) on someone else's door to get his needs met.

Stroke it to the left and stroke it to the right (brain)

Men are analytical and visual creatures. To keep him interested, you'll need to appeal to both sides. Let's start with his left brain:

Tasty Leftovers

What can you say about leftovers? You and your family probably have mixed emotions regarding them and more than likely, a family member will have strong feelings about eating them; yet, you'll find a way to fix them up-make them taste better. Similarly, when you share something with him about how you feel, he will not respond with more feelings, but with how to fix it. He'll go all around and over the subject; proceeding to take steps to fix whatever the issue is. You will need to be very direct and linear in your thinking when dealing with your man.

Men deal with facts, not feelings...hence, the right brain.

Mr. Right

Attention Girls, when dealing with your man, you will have to choose on numerous occasions aka: MOST OF THE TIME, whether you want to be right or do you want to be happy? I'm pleading with you to allow him to be right. You "settle" for happy. If you constantly argue with him, wanting to be right, you'll turn into an adversary. And it'll send a very loud message to him that you're a fighter and not his lover! This will lead to a series of silent strokes.

Stroke Symptoms

Symptoms of silent strokes will wreak havoc on your relationship. And unfortunately, you'll both experience the side effects such as:

- Trouble seeing. As in he'll stop seeing you as I said before, as his dream girl, but instead as an adversary. He will want to win-AT ALL COSTS! Winning for him will start to feel like a way to protect his manhood. If you neuter him every other day, do know, he'll start to fight for his right to have and KEEP the biggest conjones! Stop strapping on virtual dicks. Let your man have the only dick in the house.

- Sudden numbness. He'll become numb to your lack of attentiveness. He'll start pretending that it doesn't hurt.

- Sudden severe headaches. You're using the excuse of saying you have a headache in order to avoid intimacy.

- Sudden imbalance. This one is solely on you girls. Your imbalance comes from putting too much attention on things that don't matter, binging on some random television series, rather than spending quality time with your man. Which leads right into my next tip ...

STEP #3

F <u>u</u> <u>n</u> <u>d</u> HIM!

"Invest in people who invest in you"

~ unknown

I must admit, this is probably my favorite "F" him instruction.

And it has nothing to do with money.

Funding your man is to believe in him.

Is to be good to him.

To give him your most precious currency: TIME!

Relish in the time you get to be loved and the love you give to him.

Time and life are so fleeting…make every moment count.

We rarely realize this until it's too late. Usually something tragic happens to make us aware of the value of time.

"Invest in love to earn dividends of happiness." ~ Debasish Mridha

Reinvest In Your Relationship

Every really good businessman or businesswoman knows that in order to keep a business going, you must constantly reinvest profits back into the business.

Even if your marriage or union is going well, you'll still need to be cognizant of investing time and love back into the relationship. This is not the time to get sloppy or lazy and start to think that just because he's in the house on any random Saturday night, that all is well. He doesn't have to cheat seven days a week. He could be emotionally involved with someone at work or maybe that Wednesday, when he's out late, just might be the time he's being "funded" by someone else.

Strategies for Growth

You will need to constantly be looking for ways to reinvent yourself and the ways you fund the relationship. Here are a few things you should do to keep your relationship from going stale:

- Be a chameleon. Change the way you dress, your hair color and maybe lose or add weight (yes, sometimes you can be too skinny). Simply don't look the same way you did—ten years ago. Men are visual; give him something different.

- Plan a secret rendezvous. Surprise him with a hotel room key in his briefcase, toolbelt or backpack.

- Take a vacation *without* the kids.

Double Your Money

"Happiness Was Born A Twin." ~ Lord Byron

When you are happy and share that joy with your partner, you'll experience happiness twofold.

In other words, the happiness you give is the happiness you'll get.

Where some of you go wrong is thinking that if only your partner would make you happy, THEN you'd be happy!

Uh-uh honey, that is so not how this works.

You must first make yourself happy by doing whatever, and being whomever, you want to be.

I promise you, once you're singularly happy, your happiness has no choice but to become plural.

"It's an extra dividend when you like the girl you're in love with."

~ Clark Gable

Money Doesn't Grow on Trees, But Happiness Does

Happiness grows on trees?

Yes, it does.

Stay with me, Mrs. Parker.

I'm using the tree of life as a metaphor.

Think about it this way: on the tree, each branch represents a different aspect of your personality... your being. As the essence of you grows deeper, all branches will strengthen...thrive and grow. In addition, your capacity to love, become wiser or simply step into your truth, are all representative as the branches of you.

You're the tree.

And as you get taller, stronger, you "branch out" more for the world to see.

You become at peace.

And your happiness will flow outwards. Touching nearby trees.

Other people will begin to comment on how happy you two are as a couple. The world can tell you all

REALLY like one another.

Ever notice how peaceful it is to simply sit under a tree?

It's because you can feel that it's firmly rooted—maturated.

Bending with the wind.

Not fighting change…being happy.

Happy is as Happy Does

"They say a person needs just three things to be truly happy in this world: someone to love, something to do, and something to hope for." ~ Tom Bodett

Here is the interactive part of this book. Fill in the blanks of the following questions:

1. Who is your someone to love?

   _____

2. What is it that you love to do?

   _____

3. What do you hope for?

   _____

No One Wants Your Bitchcoin!

Upon waking, by making that trio of questions the inauguration of your day, you'll realize that whatever crap comes your way or whatever annoying habit your mate has, is not your business.

Focus on your own happiness and fall so in love with your own life, that annoyances become background noise. There's nothing to bitch about.

Annoyances-never too loud to distract you, but there nonetheless.

It's just part of life.

And I've found the shortcut to happiness is through the pages of your journal. While journaling, write down daily at least five things that made you smile or warmed your heart. These are great for those lonely nights or so-called bad days for reference and simply as a lil dose of happy.

"Most folks are about as happy as they make their minds up to be."

~Abraham Lincoln

STEP #4

F̲l̲l̲w̲ HIM!

"You know, you can only lead them from behind."

~ Nelson Mandela

Fllw is shorthand for follow. And I'm imploring you to follow your man.

Let him take the lead.

Give him top billing.

Let him be the face of your union.

You lead from behind.

And yes, I got some explaining to do; trust me, I'm about to do it.

I will admit, this sounds a little archaic; except this is about *seeming* to follow your man. Your man takes the lead in the outside world; by acquiescing, you lead the way where it really counts—in his heart.

So many women think it's just the opposite.

They want to make statements to everyone near and far that ain't no man gon tell them what to do-or they compete with their mates!

Good luck with that sista.

"I'm in a long term committed relationship... with my success." ~Boss Babes

Boss Babes Beware

It's all the rage (and that's a good thang) to be the boss of your own life. You're running a corporation, making your own money and buying what you want.

So much so, this Boss Babe life comes with an ad campaign:

Not only can you bring home the bacon, Fry it up in a pan.

BUT (what SOME men hear), also make him forget he was ever a man.

*All for the low, lo*w price of his manhood!

I so wish I could relay to you that most men can handle a Boss Babe.

Unfortunately, a few cannot. Those few feel as if you've slipped on their pants, strapped on and tucked a placebo penis! Their manhood feels threatened in the bedroom...and outside the bedroom. When you're too powerful, they start to feel inadequate as a man and as a provider.

So what's a Boss Babe to do?

If he can't handle you, it is not your job to 'potty train' a man into feeling better about himself or to raise his self-esteem...that's his job! And to clarify, this by no means takes away from what I just said. Those tips are based on being in a *healthy* relationship with a man who's NOT intimidated by you. Thus, if you do decide to stay—you will have to make concessions.

I've been in this situation with a couple of insecure men.

I stayed.

It didn't work.

One man in particular found his power. And exerted it...with his fists. I am not saying that your man will resort to fisticuffs. There are times though, that insecurity manifests itself in the form of verbal and mental abuse. I dated another man who just couldn't bring himself to give me a compliment-told me it'd go to my head.

Lastly, insecurity can transform into infidelity. Infidelity? Yes. He knows his adulterous ways will devastate you. You may be balling in all areas of your life, but to be cheated on-is a death blow to any woman's self-esteem.

"I find it extremely ironic that strap-on spelled backwards, spells: NO PARTS."
~unknown

What if You're Just Bossy?

Listen, it happens—you know it does.

These are the areas in which I've witnessed innumerable women of all ages, races and cultures, snatch the damn wheel and ballsacks from their men!

Restauranting

Good Lord, this is something I've seen way too often. From my days of hostessing and bartending, I've encountered so many ballsy-ass women (*pssst*... that's not a compliment.)

Nope, not at all. From the moment the couple enters the restaurant, the wife or girlfriend proceeds to take the lead.

She's first to approach the hostess.

She's the one getting up and bitching about them waiting for over an hour and how that family with the crying kids came in after them.

She's pulling up to the bar first, getting the bartender's attention, putting tip on counter beforehand (signaling she's got this), and ordering.

She's the one at the bar, playing musical chairs;

asking people to move down or switch seats to accommodate her party.

At the same time, her man or date is blasé, hanging back, and scrolling through Instagram, letting her fight these battles...lead the way.

Damn!

Really?

She orders dinner for herself...and him.

She'll tell her man what he can or cannot eat...this week they're doing Keto.

She reaches for the check FIRST!

She grabs the check to make sure that plate of slimy, overcooked brussels sprouts was taken off the tab.

If she's the wife, she'll pull out their joint debit/credit card.

If single, she pays in full...humming *Independent Women* by *Destiny's Child*.

Or she remembers that drop of Dutch blood from her ancestry test and splits the check faster than a Dutch door can open!

She determines the tip. And tip is usually based on

emotions (i.e., the server was a little too cute or flirty for her taste).

O What a Relief It Is!

"A strong man doesn't have to be dominant toward a woman. He doesn't match his strength against a woman weak with love for him. He matches it against the world."
~Marilyn Monroe

Here's the second area where we womenfolk take the lead unnecessarily: when we need some relief or resolution for a problem.

[*Back inside the restaurant*] the reason she checked the tab to make sure that plate of nasty-ass brussels sprouts was taken off, is because she'd asked that cute lil server to get the manager. And when the even *cuter* female restaurant manager came over, she was the one to bitch and demand a refund…NOT her man!

As they leave the restaurant (vowing never to return and promising to write a bad Yelp review), she proceeds to tell him how to drive.

At what speed.

In what lane.

And what route to take.

Still not convinced? Here are some more examples of bad leadership:

- On any given suburban Saturday afternoon, she's the one inside *BestBuy* showing her ass, because the price on the tag doesn't match at checkout.

- Vacays can sometimes get off to rocky starts: she's the one at the airport or hotel desk, doing the slap-her-hand-on-the-counter-pissed off routine, with a teething, drooling toddler on her hip, complaining over a booking error.

- She gets totally dragged later in the teacher lounge, after usurping the lead at any given parent/teacher conference. She's making her husband feel right at home in those tiny, red kindergarten chairs.

- Socially, she will brazenly cut her man off if she feels he isn't talking fast enough or detailing the story correctly.

- Lastly, she's *"that"* Mom at little league; yelling louder than any other mom or dad and ripping the ref and head coach a new one over her baby.

"A leader is best when people barely know he exists, when his work is done, his aim fulfilled, they will say: we did it ourselves."
~Lao Tzu

Night (gown) in Shining Armor?

A proverbial gorgeous, billowing, prima cotton night gown that some women will wear in order to protect their heart or to mask past pain.

But guess what? It doesn't have to be this way.

I promise, it's ok to let him honor you.

Protect you.

Rescue you.

Be strong enough to show weakness.

And by weakness, I mean, do not be afraid to be vulnerable.

"I don't mind living in a man's world as long as I can be a woman in it."

~ Marilyn Monroe

A lot has been said on *Facebook* about leaning in.

I'm all about taking the lead in your career, but in terms of your relationship with your man and in the words of rapper Fat Joe, "Lean back."

Allow him to be old school in his behavior (e.g., open all doors for you, pull your chair out, give you his jacket when you're cold, PAY FOR DATES, etc.)

Allow him to help you out in a financial bind.

Let him ask you to get married.

Let him fix something (small) broken in your home (even if you've *YouTubed* it and can do it).

Let him repair big appliances if he can, rather than call a professional.

Let him do the upkeep on your vehicles.

He takes the trash out.

Revel in him caring for you when ill.

Make him kill any creepy crawlers.

Delight in him getting the kids dressed and doing their hair.

Go to him for professional career advice.

Ask him his thoughts on current events.

Praise him in front of co-workers, family and neighbors after he does something special for you... as a dad, a provider.

Never refer to him as weak.

Never call him a little girl,

a bitch

or a pussy.

Never remind him that you make more money and you don't need him. Especially if he's in a blue-collar profession and you're not.

Never tell him that it's your money and you have the final say on how it's spent.

"Every man I meet wants to protect me. I can't figure out what from." ~ *Mae West*

Here's something you may not know:

Men love to rescue stuff.

And by rescue, I mean help save the day for you.

They just want to play the role of superhero in your eyes and in your life.

Let him have that.

You can give your Supergirl tee shirt a rest and allow

him to, wait for it...

LEAD THE WAY.

"A real woman can do it all by herself...but a real man won't let her."

~unknown.

Counting the Days of the Weak

In the end, if you find yourself in this situation where you MUST lead or nothing gets done, you have got to ask yourself some tough questions.

Mainly, is this the man for you?

Can you live with a man that even *allows* you to be so domineering and to act as his second mother?

I know, I know, I get it.

We as women have been checking that head of household box, running our own companies, saving Democracy (by voting in record numbers), buying homes and raising babies on our own, and some of us have forgotten how to take a backseat when it comes to dating or co-habitation.

Some older men haven't made it any easier. Many have refused to live in the twenty-first century and still behave as if it's the 1950s. Whereas, the younger generations of men are so used to things being handed to them, with no clue how to even be a real man and/or biding by the "everybody wins mentality," it's no wonder so many women are confused.

For me it's very simple—I NEED A STRONG MAN.

And by strong, I mean:

- A man who has enough respect for himself wouldn't dream of letting me disrespect him in the home or outside the home.

- A man who will not allow me to pay for our dinner and drinks when initially dating; he appreciates and recognizes that I am the prize.

- A strong man who, when shit gets rough, does what needs to be done to take care of his family and responsibilities. And if that meant getting multiple jobs—he wouldn't hesitate.

- A man that appreciates my entrepreneurial desires and encourages me to follow all my crazy ideas and dreams.

- A man that isn't scared to say I love you and express his emotions. Likewise, he isn't afraid to show vulnerability and/or cry in front of me.

- A man that tells me the truth…even when it hurts.

- A man that will call bullshit when I deserve it.

- A man who isn't threatened by my beauty, nor jealous of me and my accomplishments.

- A man that mentally challenges me.

- A man that I can debate and exchange sexy banter with-*with ease!*

- And most importantly, a man that respects my womanhood— however I define it.

- A man who would never call me a derogatory name or resort to physical or emotional violence to exert control. He'd leave the relationship before resorting to such behavior.

This is a man that I would follow anywhere...because I trust in him as a leader and I trust that he wouldn't lead me astray.

Which makes me want to...

STEP #5

F u c k HIM!

"Sex is like air; it's not important unless you aren't getting any."

~John Callahan

Ahhh, what you *really* thought this book was going to be all about.

Ladies, sex is duct tape for anything broken in your relationship.

It'll hold it together, until you figure it out!

HeadBoard Honcho

You are in charge in the bedroom. Your best position?

Be on top…of your game!

We as women are always in charge of how a relationship will go.

Men want to please us; and if you express your needs to him, he will work overtime to fulfill them. In turn, you get the pleasure of repaying him with the gift that produces great dividends (those damn dividends again), for you as well!

Every time you make love to him, kiss him, or hold him, you are solidifying his love for you.

Give Head

"THINGS YOU NEVER HEAR: "Please stop sucking my dick or I'll call the police." ~George Carlin

And yet, that's not the head I'm referring to.

Nope.

Girls, get in his head, before and after you get in and out the bed.

You will need to make love to his

manhood

his pride

his ego

and to his soul.

Kiss Him, You Fool!

"A kiss is a secret told to the mouth instead of the ear; kisses are the messengers of love and tenderness." ~Ingrid Bergman

And I mean a real kiss!

Kiss that man on the lips.

None of that side cheek shit.

Save that for your dad, brother or male friends. But your man-he needs to connect with you physically. Before he leaves the house and when he returns home, give him a long, wet kiss on the lips. And especially when making love, invite your tongue in on the action.

Kissing is very intimate. And very IMPORTANT! I promise you, kissing is the telltale sign to measuring the health of a relationship. If kissing him on the mouth makes you queasy-something is off.

Remember the *Pretty Woman* mantra: no kissing on the lips. It wasn't until she (Julia Roberts) fell for Richard Gere's character, that she allowed herself to open up and get intimate with him with a fullthroated, tongue-all-down-his throat kiss.

"People have forgotten what the human touch is, what it is to smile, for somebody to smile at them, somebody to recognize them, somebody to wish them well. The terrible thing is to be unwanted." ~Mother Teresa

Rub One Out

Rub his back...stroke him...nurture him.

Touch him often.

Make him feel wanted...desired.

According to *Psychology Today*, babies who are not held, nuzzled, and hugged enough can stop growing, and if the situation lasts long enough, even die.

Girls, please don't let your relationship with your baby daddy, boo thang, or bae, die.

Give that man a damn hug!

In addition, he will need you to love him for him. Never try to change him. Love him completely for who he is, what he stands for, and his truth.

Most importantly, love and support his dreams.

Encourage him to be a

better man

citizen

father

and earthling.

Fuck Him Up!

Yes girl, fuck him up.

Wake him up to fuck in the morning,

fuck him in the afternoon,

and fuck him at night.

Fuck when he wants to and when you want to.

Fuck him every day.

Work overtime not to reject his advances.

And I am not here for the excuses!

Expand your thoughts on what it means to "fuck."

Remember all those torrid, spontaneous lovemaking sessions you two had in the beginning? You didn't think about scheduling sex, it just flowed naturally. Intimacy reared its beautiful head in numerous forms. There was a togetherness that went beyond the physical…you two were connected spiritually…energetically. But now that the euphoria is fading, 'ain't nothing going on but the rent', and there may or may not be children in the house, figure out a way to connect with him physically on some level. Some days it just may be a hot and heavy make out session. A series of sexy sexts. A shower together.

Hand holding on a long walk. Eye contact held over drinks. One of the sexiest things I've ever seen was when the late JFK Jr. looked at his beautiful bride, Caroline Bessette-Kennedy, and kissed the back of her hand while looking directly into her eyes. That, my friends is intimacy. I'm grown enough to know that love making begins way before your legs are in the air.

"You know that look women get when they want to have sex? Yeah, me neither."

~ Steve Martin

Anytime I hear a man joke openly about can/or will he get some from his wife, that's probably because she has gotten real stingy with it (there's always truth in humor).

And only you can answer that question as to why.

Why don't you enjoy making love to your husband?

Is he a bad lover?

Does having sex trigger a bad memory and/or traumatic event for you?

Are you hormonal?

Have you shared your concerns?

If none of the above pertains to you, then miss me with all that you're screaming into these pages right now. Admit it Honey, you're claiming to be tired, simply to get out of having sex with him—for whatever reason.

Where has the thrill gone?

Why has it gone underground or off the grid?

Figure that shit out.

Especially if you're a *healthy* woman. Or married to a wealthy man who absolutely adores you and provides you with a very easy lifestyle complete with housekeepers and nannies! Maybe you're the breadwinner; clearly, you're used to climbing that proverbial corporate ladder, so why have you stopped climbing into bed with your man?

I will give my working and single moms, without all the trappings of the rich, a slight break—but even you need to keep fanning those flames OFTEN.

But if the hardest thing you do all day is a hot yoga class and wait in line in your tricked out mini-van or Range Rover to pick up your kids from an exclusive private school, then (and I say this with love), Oh hell no, Sweetie-get to fucking!

Are You a SexPot?

Ok, this is so not going where you think it's going. This isn't about how sexy you feel or if you play dress up with your man. No, you're way off. I'm asking: do you need weed, aka marijuana, pills or alcohol to get emotionally undressed, and to have and/or enjoy sex with your man?

And this is where I'll need pure, unadulterated honesty from you.

Sharing is caring.

Let's recap, shall we?

Do you remember in my intro, I touched upon needing a drink? Well, more like several cosmopolitans to be exact (hey it was the 90s; all the gals on *Sex and The City* were drinking them) and this was my 'cool-aid.' Those vodka-laced drinks aided and abetted me in my arousal plans operation honey trap. It was like having a

Ménage-a-trois

O yes, Honey, I welcomed a sexy Russian brewed, dulcet, full-bodied, pink-hued lady-of-the-night into my crumbling marital bed, two to three times a week.

And she was so good.

For about eighteen minutes, her vodka kisses silenced my apathy; she soothed my open wounds...coating my emotional pain. She was very seductive and used her magical pheromones to liquify my inhibitions, fire up my desire, seduce my husband and most importantly, she skillfully used her talents as an agent provocateur to put all my problems to sleep... if only for the night.

Afternoon Delight?

Oh no, I wouldn't dare try to have sex during the day—you're kidding right? Day drinking (heavily) probably would've blown my cover-unless we were on vacation. And as for kissing and touching, I was quite curmudgeonly. I was at times literally revulsed.

I pulled away from him often and avoided kissing him on the mouth.

I tried and failed, in the end, to use her 40% proof to make my marriage divorce proof.

Am I proud? No. Am I honest? Yes.

I'm willing to bet and go all the way to the end of the limb-I am not alone.

My numbing agent was alcohol-what's yours?

When we're not happy, most emotionally unaware people will turn to something else to make whatever the situation may be, much more palatable. This can rear its mutated head in forms such as abusing food, drugs and alcohol, to excessive shopping, working and even Bible studying...*hello*-Jesus Freaks!

"Avoiding problems you need to face, is avoiding life you need to live."

~Paulo Coelho

Mr. Sensitivity

Men are extremely sensitive! Men make love to show exactly how much they care for us. Too much rejection from you will cause him to withdraw. And when he withdraws from you, he will be *drawn* to another woman!

(Hey, don't get mad at me—I'm just the messenger.)

That's right, when his executive assistant or cute co-worker who *oohs* and *ahhs* over him, is telling him daily how smart he is, she will start to look like a damn supermodel in his eyes. And not that he wants to have an affair—he's simply needy, lonely and hungry as hell...starving emotionally for attention!

And if he starts taking her to lunch--you in trouble, girl.

Sex with another woman is inevitable.

And this is when being the only dick in the house takes on a negative connotation.

American Express Pink Card (never let him leave home without it!)

Translation: don't ever let your man leave the house without his pink card issued by the bank of you.

He's been a member since whatever year you all started dating. He will never need to borrow or use anyone else's pink card. Why? Because the sky's the limit- he has unlimited charging privileges! And not necessarily in just sex.

Back Door Shenanigans!

Relax...unclench those cheeks, it's not what you're thinking.

Do not leave your back door open for a second!

I'll explain.

If you don't give your man what he craves and desires emotionally, if he starts to feel lonely, he will creep out the back door-or some chick will be checking to see if you got him on lockdown.

And if that door ain't locked, she will slip through the smallest crack!

And just so we're all very clear: MEN DO NOT GO WITHOUT SEX!

You may not have sex with him for over six months, but trust and believe, he's having sex— with someone else.

Ask yourself this: do you want a husband or a

wasband? As in, he *was* your husband.

So, while you're sitting in the house, all in your feelings, with your legs double crossed, keep this in mind:

"Women need a reason to have sex.

Men just need a place."

~ Billy Crystal

STEP #6

F r e e HIM!

> *"When a man is denied freedom to live the life he believes in, he has no choice but to become an outlaw."*
>
> *~ Nelson Mandela*

You cannot

control,

dictate,

dominate your mate's time,

nor deny him the right to be his own man.

In other words: give your man the freedom to play golf on the weekends, go fishing, play video games, play a musical instrument, watch every sport on every single cable channel, mobile app and pay per view that he wants. And if you can afford it, rejoice in him getting season tickets to his favorite team, six months in advance!

Do not control his hobbies,

how much he eats or drinks,

or anything that relaxes him.

You are not his mother. You are his lover.

And if you want to keep the fire burning like a Texas bonfire for years, build that damn mancave-

JUST FOR HIM!

It shall not double as the kids' playroom or where your book club meets once a month.

Miss me on the scolding, side-eye shade and the counting of his beers.

Go do you!

Go do some shit inside your she shed.

He may be your best friend, but he ain't your buddy.

Go get you some buddies and get off his back.

For if you don't, there wil be consequences.

Translation: He'll start to sneak and do the things he wants to do.

And lie.

Which in turn, will piss you off; aka—hurt you.

And just like that, the prisoner has staged a revolt-a

prison riot.

All for a simple weekend furlough.

Girls, let me be very clear once again. I am not saying he gets to ignore his duties as a dad or as a husband. I'm saying whatever he likes to do in his free time—let him! And no, if it's harmful to his health, that's an entirely different subject. But if he likes to play band with his middle-aged rocker boys, let him. If he likes to smoke a lil greenery and you hate it—oh well. A wife with an attitude about something she hates should not affect a husband's ability to indulge.

"Freedom is not worth having if it doesn't include the right to make mistakes."

~ Mahatma Gandhi

Your man will make mistakes.

I repeat: Your man will make mistakes!

Your man is not perfect, and I promise you, he will make numerous mistakes in

loving you,

in his duties as a dad

and as a provider.

Therefore...

STEP #7

F <u>giv</u> HIM!

> ***"There is no revenge so complete as forgiveness."***
>
> ***~Josh Billings***

Yes, this is text talk for FORGIVE.

FORGIVE HIM, GIRLS!

For those who have watched *Sex & The City* (clearly as much as I did), back when it originally aired or on re-runs, you may recall after Carrie had cheated with Mr. Big and Aiden found out, Carrie begged Aiden to forgive her. She knew for them to move on and try to love each other again, he had to forgive her. And that's not only true for our favorite fictional characters, but this is a fact, though it may seem just as strange as fiction.

"When you forgive, you in no way change the past - but you sure do change the future."
~Bernard Meltzer

Let's be very clear, I'm not saying to justify his actions nor overlook them. But if he is worth keeping and what he did isn't serial and/or illicit, gravely illegal or self—destructive behavior, then give that man another chance.

Forgive him for hurting you, having an affair (this is a tough one and I'm not condoning nor condemning any decision you make that's best for you), or if something less serious, such as forgetting your wedding anniversary.

But before I go any further, I would be remiss if I did not spend a little more time on cheating.

"Most people cheat because they're paying more attention to what's missing rather than to what they have."

~unknown

How does one get over that?

Not easily, that's for damn sure!

I will not justify his improprieties by blaming you for his actions.

In the end, he ALWAYS HAS A CHOICE.

I'm just acknowledging that men don't do a lot of thinking with their big heads; their small heads tend to take over.

Most people lack the emotional maturity needed to have bare-bone honest, legitimate conversations with their mates about their unmet needs.

Especially men.

Men are extremely vulnerable—but they don't like to show it. We as moms and dads actually encourage our little boys to be so-called "big boys" and dry those tears. The impact of that message haunts them for a lifetime. Our little boys and soon-to-be adult men translate showing emotions, trying to tell someone, "It hurts," and crying as weak. So fast forward twenty-five years, that little boy is now married; his wife is rejecting him, he's feeling some sense of inadequacy in his career, his feelings get hurt daily and rather than verbalize his feelings, he doesn't talk

AT ALL—he simply bucks up, holds back the tears and goes and gets laid.

It's easier.

It damn sho' ain't weakness (in his mind).

It's familiar...comfy.

Can I digress for a second? I'm always shocked that people are more comfy with getting undressed and having sex with new partners, than getting emotionally naked and talking about their sexual needs with someone they love.

That person who is their in-case-of-emergency/next of kin.

The beneficiary on their life insurance policy.

Someone who has all their numbers: social security, sleep and bank accounts.

Those with whom they share parenting duties.

In my opinion, humans are petrified to go down this rabbit hole of honesty. Lord knows, all kinds of secrets are buried deep down there. They just might have to face the brutally ugly truth in other areas of their life.

As a result, that hurting husband of yours will be drawn to a hurt little girl...masking as a grown-ass woman (like attracts like). A woman whose heart has been broken one too many times-from a smorgasbord of pain—pick one:

- Daddy issues
- Abuse in any of its nasty forms
- Heartaches
- Self-esteem or lack thereof

But most significantly, he'll meet a lonely woman. A woman that simply wants to pretend to be loved... held.

They'll bond through their shared pain and ravenous appetite for human touch.

In no way am I saying that it's right, vindicated... exculpated. But I am willing to look deeper, to understand.

To not judge it too harshly.

Because what I know for sure-*nothing* is out of order!

No experience goes wasted...your mess can end up being a blessing for you or someone later.

Everything that happens is for a reason.

And that's for all parties involved to figure out.

Oh, and that lonely woman...I know her very well.

I was once her.

"The best apology is changed behavior."
~unknown

If you choose to take your partner back after an affair, you have got to live in the now and not stay stuck in the past.

The only thing that the past is good for is learning from it.

Otherwise, visiting the past is a waste of time.

How to recognize you aren't living in the now: can you get in your car and put in directions to go back to that sunny Tuesday, July 10th, 2007 at approximately 12:39pm. Location: Miami Beach, *Wet Willies* bar? Um, the last time I checked, that Tesla guy hadn't invented this car yet!

Therefore, since you can't go there physically, why are you choosing to go there every day ONLY in your mind? It's not real anymore. But when you constantly go back reliving that painful experience, you keep giving that memory life.

It's not real.

You can't change the past.

Stop it...please.

"Without forgiveness, there's no future."
~Desmond Tutu

Back To The Future

Where I *do* encourage you to go and visualize in your mind-to the future!

Yes, that's right, I need you to constantly see yourself loving him and enjoying yourself again with him.

Your new thoughts will create a new future.

See it the way you want it to be.

"A happy marriage is the union of two good forgivers."

~Ruth Graham

BONUS TIP

F o o l HIM

NOT!!!!

"My fake plants died because I did not pretend to water them."

~Mitch Hedberg

Just in case you don't remember my most dire warning in my opening statement, then let me remind you: I married a man that I loved on some level, but a man that I did not respect. And in the beginning, I fooled myself, thinking that I could live like this.

Turns out—not so much.

I knew I married the wrong man about three days after our courthouse wedding. It became even more clear when I found myself needing a cocktail before I had sex.

I knew this inner turmoil could not be sustained.

I knew that I would one: end up an alcoholic.

Or two:

I would simply stop having sex with him.

Well hell, I was married and that wasn't fair to him.

I said this at the beginning, and I feel obligated to say it again: the only reason I am divulging this much information about my former marriage, again, is NOT to sell books, or throw my 'wasbend' under the bus; but to really drive home my point and to let you know, I'm preaching from experience:

You cannot fool a man.

If you don't like him or if you really don't love him, guess who'll give you away?

No, not your jealous-much girlfriend who always liked him. You know the one, the one you don't trust alone in the kitchen with him.

Oh no, it'll be YOU!

That's right,

your body

your spirit

your attitude

and your nerves will respond to him exactly how you subconsciously feel about him...

Repulsed.

"I can't get married. I can't fake sleep for 30 years."

~Elayne Boosler

Marriage is not to be taken lightly.

And you damn sure can't fake a good one.

But oh, how some of you will try.

Try as some of you might,

we can all see a fake good marriage coming at us a mile away.

You're that couple that stopped having sex…years ago.

You're that couple in which one or both are having not-so-secret affairs.

You're that couple that rarely takes vacations alone- always with other couples.

You're that couple that argues in front of other people…on said vacations.

You're that couple that boozes it up way too much at dinner parties.

You're that couple walking on eggshells around each other.

You're that couple that talks shit about your spouse and teases them relentlessly under the guise of, "just joking."

You're that couple we all feel so uncomfortable around. We witness cracks in the foundation—in real time.

You're that couple that actually fights one another! Usually the man has stab wounds, the wife-bruises to prove it. You two are legendary in your neighborhood and at family reunions.

You're that couple still putting on Oscar-worthy performances at social functions and corporate events-pretending to be that happy couple.

You're that couple that seems to have it all:

Wealth

Vacation homes

Well-behaved children

Societal standing

And yet...

You're that couple that we took $10 bets on that you'll never divorce; versus, we give it six months to a year. The pot is over $5000.

It's *War of the Roses*...2.0

Sorry, but if one or more of these apply you're *that* couple.

Don't be that couple.

Make-A-Wish Foundation

And that's my hope for you. To lay the foundation of your relationship with your greatest wish. That wish for that great love you've always dreamed of. We all know when we're going through the motions of day-to-day life. We know when our hearts are yearning for more. We know when we're married to the lifestyle, rather than to the man. I am such a believer in mind, body and spirit; that is why I know when you're not living your truth or with your true love-physical signs will mysteriously emerge, and your spirits will be low.

"Let each know that for each the body, the mind and the soul have been freed to fulfill themselves."

~Nelson Mandela

You must begin telling yourself the truth...the truth will always set you free.

"At every crossroads on the path that leads to the future, tradition has placed 10,000 men to guard the past."

~Maurice Maeterlinck

F <u>A</u> <u>C</u> <u>E</u> the Truth

WARNING: IT'S GONNA GET HOPE UP IN HERE!

Yes, I know you were expecting "hot" rather than "hope"—ME TOO! But the universe had other plans. My hands seem to type on their own and I'm gonna roll with it.

I sincerely *hope* that one day, more couples will have those much-needed, extraordinarily painful, yet therapeutic and revealing, and once joked about, conscious uncoupling conversations.

Ms. Gwyneth was ahead of her time.

Imagine discovering your husband wasn't happy and/or was having an affair. And rather than get mad—you set him free. Because you knew deep down that you did not and could not give him the passion and love he deserved...and what you deserved! We all deserve to live a passionate, zestful life.

What if you stepped outside your ego and didn't look at it as the other woman winning or you as losing- but as a vehicle to move forward to a better life for you and him.

It's just a thought and wishful thinking...for most

people aren't this woke.

Unfortunately, the majority of egos are too fragile for this level of truth.

"Let us not seek to satisfy our thirst for freedom by drinking from the cup of bitterness and hatred."

~Martin Luther King, Jr.

When you aren't living your highest self and by doing so-feeling free, you will inevitably act out. Acting out shows up in a plethora of ways: road rage, thoughts of suicide, irritability, oversensitivity, overeating and a truck load of ism's: alcoholism, hyperthyroidism, and criticism to name a few. I could go on naming an entire manuscript of *dis- eases* that will show up. But that's when you got to slip outta those cute lil thongs and put your big girl panties on.

Stop lying to yourself!

If the partner you have in your life has stopped growing with you and/or is past their season, DO EVERYTHING IN YOUR POWER TO MAKE IT RIGHT. Talk to them, see if things can change and if not, go make yourself happy. And yes, that may mean divorce, breaking up your family or moving on.

Otherwise, you really will live up to that vow of "till death do you part."

A slow…painful…daily death—on repeat! Everyday a part of you will die a little death. Making you a very lonely, unhappy woman.

I find it very ironic that society praises long-term marriages. EVEN if the man has been unfaithful, had children out of wedlock, or emotionally abuses his wife!

> *"In a bad marriage, friends are the invisible glue. If we have enough friends, we may go on for years, intending to leave, talking about leaving - instead of actually getting up and leaving."*
>
> *~Erica Jong*

Maybe the onus is on you-you've simply outgrown him. You two are not happy! And yet, the ladies you lunch with encourage you to stay-telling you it doesn't matter, at least you're married!

It's such a subtle way of saying to women: that it's better to be married than to be alone.

Personal growth and happiness take a backseat to a joint tax return.

I simply don't buy into the idea of the widely held belief that marriage is hard. I stop my married girlfriends from even saying that phrase. Don't put that out into the universe—the universe LOVES to make you a martyr! I believe the only time marriage is hard, is when one or both partners have settled for less in some shape, form, or fashion.

And let me state this without any misunderstandings, I am NOT saying you won't have any challenges. Of course, you will...shit happens. But going home every night after work shouldn't make you feel dread or look for an excuse to work late.

In other words, if this is how you feel, then you're not being authentic to your true desires.

Be ok with change, if every rock has been turned

over and therapy has been sought. You deserve to be a happy, joyful woman that thoroughly enjoys f _ _ _ing (tip #5) her man.

But one last thing...

For F_ _ k's Sake, NEVER FORSAKE HIM!

Fight fairly!

Never throw out the "D" word unless you seriously plan on doing it, got a retainer fee in hand and an appointment with a divorce attorney. So many of us will scream to our man, *"I want a divorce!"* so cavalierly, while simply having a very heated argument, when, *"I'm really pissed off right now!"* would have sufficed.

If you always threaten to leave or to divorce him, that sends strong signals back to him, that he cannot trust you to stick around when the going gets rough and that it's an all or nothing sum game with you.

In other words-you're an emotional terrorist!

You rejoice in desecrating the entire household, keeping him and your kids teetering on an emotional highwire. More than that, you resort to extreme measures (e.g., packing up your belongings and children and disappearing for a few days or giving him the silent treatment for weeks—and him not knowing when you'll attack again). All this purely to exact payback, and to get or have things go your way—AT ALL COSTS!

Every time you engage in terroristic behavior by threatening divorce, it's like dropping an atomic bomb in your living room.

Fallout, mass destruction be damned!

Congrats—you're the newest housewife on The Real Housewives of Isis!

But be very careful—as I'm sure you've watched one of the Real Housewives franchises, your so-called friends and friendly fire can be a bitch.

"Divorce isn't such a tragedy. A tragedy's staying in an unhappy marriage, teaching your children the wrong things about love. Nobody ever died of divorce."

~Jennifer Weiner

"When two people decide to get a divorce, it isn't a sign that they 'don't understand' one another, but a sign that they have, at least, begun to."

~Helen Rowland

"Heartbreak is a loss. Divorce is a piece of paper."

~Taylor Jenkins Reid

EAT shit, PRAY that you die & Love every minute of it!

Elizabeth Gilbert never went into too much detail about her personal feelings towards her first husband, but I wager you—she had them (and was all in'em) AND she probably echoed my sentiments at some point but kept it much classier in her book: *Eat, Pray, Love.* All jokes aside, every woman I know that has had to undergo a painful separation has uttered some demented version of this statement, while ugly crying with her bestie after receiving a terse letter from her soon-to-be ex's divorce attorney. The letters tend to inform her about money, the house, the kids or what he plans on keeping. And she usually reads and re-reads them several times, while death clutching a big, overflowing glass of an adult beverage.

I can tell you firsthand that divorce is a bitch!

I know it from all sides:

- As a child: I saw my parents fight both verbally and physically; eventually enduring the antics of a brutal separation. It came to a head one night, which involved a sleezy 70s motel, busted out windows of a brown 1975 Fleetwood Cadillac and my pregnant mother. It would make for a helluva movie scene!

- As a wife: I went through my own ugly unraveling of the "dream."
- As a friend: I've been there helping my friends navigate those choppy waters.

In some ways, divorce is like death and all its surreal stages.

Except, your ignorant-ass ex ain't dead.

Nope, not at all.

He's living in the city, in a tricked-out bachelor pad with killer views, bangin' twenty-year olds, and has had the nerve to lose 30 pounds!

And not that you want him back, but you feel all alone…old.

While he seems to be living his best dad bod life!

No worries. Stop snacking on those chewy cuticles.

He ain't happy…he's busy.

Busy avoiding his feelings for you.

But this too shall pass.

In the meantime, you can't despise your ex—no matter what he did or said. You must always have more love and respect for yourself and/or your children, than hate for him.

So, in the end, do what's best for both parties.

Do it with love.

Have no F <u>e</u> <u>a</u> <u>r</u>...

Flee HIM!

Thanks for coming to my ~~TED~~ SPREAD TALK!

(Sexual Perspectives Revealed, Expressed And Discussed)

Ideas worth spreading

I sincerely hope you've enjoyed my little book about how to "F" your man.

Everything I shared with you either came naturally or I did the legs-in-the-air work.

I've been a huge fan of men for some time.

All my life, even as I played with my Barbie dolls, I would fantasize about a great love. A great love that was all encompassing and that would last a lifetime. I, like other girls and maybe you, yearned for that fairytale love.

I finally found it.

No not with a man,

but with myself.

I finally discovered that the great love I cherished, was the love I needed to give to myself!

All the f_ _ _ing in the world, would never feel as good as the love I give to myself numerous times a day.

I'm an insatiable for some Velicia...I love me some me!

And the only thing I need from men

nowadays are three lil letters: *ier*

That's right, I only need men to make me *happier,* because I'm already happy. *Wealthier,* because I want a man to bring his wealth of life experience and richness to my life. And lastly, *prettier*—to brighten my days with his beautiful soul.

Over the years, I've had the privilege of making love to some super sweet, broke ass guys and some phenomenally accomplished men. I've shared the sheets with a Superbowl MVP, a rock star, CEOs of billionaire corporations and tech giants, With my innate desires, skills and the practiced implementations of the aforementioned steps, these men spoiled me with lavish gifts, bucket-list vacations, cars, money and a few proposals. And I say privilege, because all these men allowed me to pick their brains.

I am completely fascinated by people who achieve greatly.

AND those that underperform...we all have a story.

I'm like a detective, searching for inspiration and tips...for success *always* leaves clues!

Even the financially challenged guys who had nothing to share but themselves, had big dreams that they wanted to pursue. And I reveled in being their head cheerleader.

In retrospect, my inquisitiveness and curiosity were probably a turn-on.

An ego booster.

I was/am childlike in my questioning.

I wanted to know about them as little boys, teenagers and what makes them tick,

how they trained,

what they ate,

who raised them

and what books they read.

I studied them…and they studied me (that's why I felt so confident in writing this book).

All that mutual studying was very seductive.

Our beds were like proverbial petri dishes.

I earned their trust.

They knew I would never kiss and tell.

I just tell tales about those kisses…

but that's a whole other book.

The End

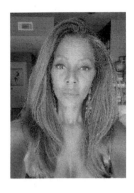 **Velicia Hill** is a former professional runway model, an Emmy winner, and the founder & Editor-In-Chief of Ms. Heel Magazine. She's currently running around in 5-inch heels in and around Hollywood...of the South.

You can follow her on Instagram

@veliciahill or veliciahill.com

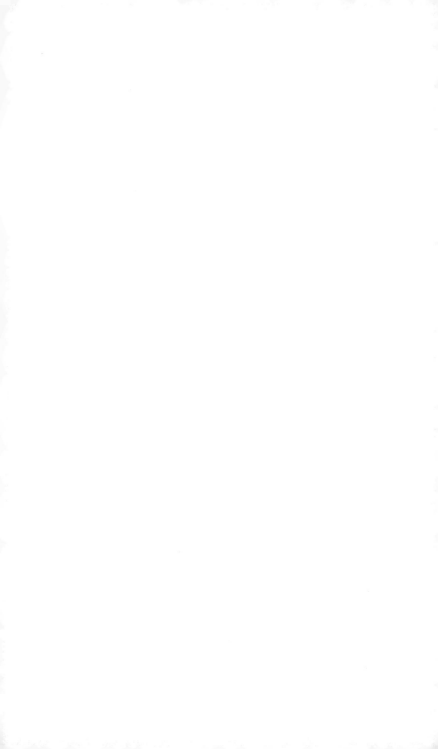

Made in the USA
Middletown, DE
28 December 2022